Apple Cider Vinegar:

101 Apple Cider Vinegar Cures, Uses And Recipes For Health, Beauty And Weight Loss

By Alicia Hern

© Copyright 2016 by Alicia Hern- All rights reserved.

It is illegal to reproduce, transmit or duplicate any part of this document through any printing or electronic means. Recording or duplication of this publication is strictly prohibited by law as well as any storage of this document, unless there is written consent on the part of the intellectual property rights holder. All rights reserved.

The author and/or intellectual property rights holder is not to be held liable for any of the information used or misused in this book. Anyone who uses or misuses the information contained within this e-book does so at their own risk. If any health issues or other problems result the author and/or intellectual property rights holder is not to be held liable for the said problem. If the information is used by anyone reading this book, the person should understand it is entirely at his/her own discretion and thereby relieving the author of any responsibility.

Disclaimer

Talk with your doctor first. Before you begin using any new health product or start a new health regimen, consult your physician to ensure that there are no risks of that product interfering with current medications, agitating current illnesses, or posing a health risk in any way.

Table Of Contents

Chapter 1. Benefits of Apple Cider Vinegar

Chapter 2. Apple Cider Vinegar for Weight Loss

Chapter 3. Beauty Recipes

Chapter 4. Detoxing

Chapter 5. Breakfast, Lunch, Dinner, Salads and Salad Dressings

Chapter 6. Natural Cures Healing the Body of Disorders

CONCLUSION

Introduction

An apple a day keeps the doctor away, and so does a daily dose of apple cider vinegar. Apple cider vinegar is a type of vinegar made from apples and has a characteristic amber color. That bottle of apple cider vinegar in your kitchen cabinet is capable of so much more than adding flavor to a salad. In fact, it may be time to move it to the medicine cabinet. Organic apple cider vinegar is antibacterial, antiviral and antifungal, so it can soothe your sore throat, heal your heartburn, remove that persistent wart and so much more. Plus, it's all natural and inexpensive.

If you knew of a product that had been around for centuries, promoted by famous physicians and scholars, consumed by armies for boosting strength and maintaining the health of soldiers, utilized on battlegrounds for its healing properties, was even mentioned in the Bible, and had hundreds of health benefits that were well documented, would you want it? Of course you would! Imagine that this amazing all-natural product could be purchased right in your local grocery store for only a few dollars.

Every day, more and more people are turning to homeopathic, natural alternatives to the modern medicines that are prescribed for everything from a bee sting to the common cold. After all, many of these modern medicines deemed "safe" for over-the-counter sale come packed with harmful chemicals, possibly dangerous additives, and a host of possible side effects. Sure, they might work, but at what cost to your body?

Skip the pharmacy aisle and instead grab apple cider vinegar—an easy-to-find, simple-to-use, safe, all-natural, age-old solution that is well known for its reputation and effectiveness.

That's right—apple cider vinegar is a simplistic answer to so many of the minor and major woes we all experience. It's not a magical, expensive, or hard-to-get, celebrity-endorsed product that is advertised or skillfully marketed to the masses—it's an inexpensive product that is all-natural and has decades of support from both consumers and science.

Which apple cider vinegar should I buy?

Apple cider vinegar is not to be confused with the regular, white vinegar found in most kitchens. White vinegar is used in cooking, as well as an effective cleaner in the kitchen, bathroom, and for washing. White vinegar, however, is refined and does not have the health benefits of apple cider vinegar.

Let's look at the top brands which are both reliable, and easy on your wallet.

Bragg

As one of the oldest brands of apple cider vinegar in the market, Bragg is also one of the most trusted brands to buy. Based on my survey (see the survey at the end of this article), most of my readers have voted for Bragg.

The California-based company says that 100% of its apples are sourced from within the United States. Because of this, they have better control of their quality. They use organic apples only, and claim that they're free from arsenic and pesticides. They also claim to use wooden barrels, which "boosts its natural fermentation qualities."

Founded by Paul C. Bragg, who was an advisor to many Olympians, the brand is now supported by Paul's daughter and nutritionist Dr. Patricia Bragg.

Vitacost

While Bragg is specifically known for its apple cider vinegar range, Vitacost is a widely known company for health products in general. Apple cider vinegar is just one of the products they sell.

In fact, Vitacost is also a retailer of other brands of vinegar that include Bragg and Dynamic Health.

Vitacost claims that their apple cider vinegar is the fermented juice of fresh-pressed 100% organic apples. It is unpasteurized, and contains the "mother," the "nutrient-rich sediment responsible for the amber/brown color and cloudy, string-like appearance of natural apple cider vinegar." There's no added sugar, artificial flavors and colors. Also, it is kosher and suitable for vegetarians.

If you are looking for cheaper but quality brand, then Vitacost is an option to consider.

Fleischmann's

You can also consider buying Fleischmann's apple cider vinegar. California-based Fleischmann began making vinegar in the 1920s when they decided to use the alcohol produced by the bakers' yeast growth.

With advances in technology, the production of bakers' yeast reduced the production of alcohol. They then entered the specialty vinegar business.

Dynamic Health

Founded in 1994, Dynamic Health provides a range of health supplements and products which are kosher, halal-certified, organic, and are available in liquid as well as capsule form.

Dynamic Health's apple cider vinegar is price competitive, but they give you a great value for the money.

Chapter 1. Benefits of Apple Cider Vinegar

The beauty of the apple cider vinegar production process is that the amazing health benefits of apples remain intact. The key is to buy raw, unfiltered apple cider vinegar—that's the kind that's cloudy. Because of the careful process by which raw, undiluted apple cider vinegar is created, the essential nutrients that are so sought after remain intact and unadulterated. Apples are packed with vitamins and minerals, which give ACV its myriad health benefits. Here are the minerals present and their health benefits:

- Potassium: muscle contraction, nerve impulses, and energy production
- Calcium: important for bone health
- Copper: nerve functioning, bone maintenance, proper utilization of glucose
- Iron: transport of oxygen, blood health
- Chromium: regulating blood glucose
- Magnesium: synthesis of proteins, cellular energy production
- Manganese: formation and maintenance of bone, carbohydrate metabolism
- Selenium: antioxidant properties, fat metabolism
- Sodium: maintains proper fluid balance
- Zinc: promotes healing
- Phosphorous: proper cell functioning, strong bones

In addition to that impressive list of minerals, there are also a number of essential vitamins found in ACV:

- Vitamin A: eye health, powerful antioxidant
- Vitamin C: immune system functioning, powerful antioxidant
- Vitamin E: skin, nerve health; powerful antioxidant

- Vitamin B1: nervous system functioning, digestive health, muscle health
- Vitamin B2: promotes healthy skin, hair, and nails; aids in breakdown of proteins, carbs, and fats
- Vitamin B12: red blood cell formation, proper nerve cell functioning
- Vitamin B6: alleviates skin conditions and nerve damage, assists in utilization of proteins, carbs, and fats

Apples (and apple cider vinegar) also contain pectin, which has been shown to aid in digestion. That's how ACV is able to act as a cleansing agent and assist the colon in ridding the body of toxins and waste that have built up over time. The pectin in ACV forms a gel-like substance that makes debris easier to move in the digestive system so it gets carried away ... naturally.

The "Mother" in Apple Cider Vinegar

If the long list of vitamins and minerals wasn't enough to impress, apple cider vinegar also contains the all-powerful "mother." "Mother" is the cobweb-like or sediment-like substance that can be seen floating in the unfiltered varieties of ACV. The mother contains the concentrated bacteria and enzymes that give ACV the antifungal, antiviral, and antibacterial healing powers for which it has become so famous. While some people may be caught off-guard by the sediment in their ACV bottles, this element is the result of the specific processing that retains the nutrients and enzymes of the apples throughout the fermentation process that provides the healing powers unique to ACV.

Are ACV Supplements Just as Beneficial?

You can also find ACV in supplement form in the vitamin aisle at your local pharmacy. While the supplement companies who produce this product claim that the benefits are the same as using ACV in its natural state, there is little research corroborating that. The truth is that while supplement manufacturers claim the potency of their products to be true, there is no real way of knowing what each tablet contains, how it's made, or the safety of consuming it. (Unlike medicines, the U.S. Food and Drug Administration doesn't regulate supplements.)

On the contrary, liquid ACV is produced by reputable companies who have been in the business of ACV production for years and are fervent advocates of their product's safety and effectiveness. While it may seem easier to swallow a tablet, the dangers of the supplement version are proven; in one specific case, a consumer suffered serious esophageal damage when an apple cider vinegar tablet became stuck in her throat. The acidic foundation of ACV makes a supplement potentially harmful. When you dilute the liquid form, you're eliminating that hazard.

Apple cider vinegar is not to be confused with the regular, white vinegar found in most kitchens. White vinegar is used in cooking, as well as an effective cleaner in kitchen, bathroom, and for washing. White vinegar, however, is refined and does not have the health benefits of apple cider vinegar.

A Few Caveats

After reading about the amazing benefits of apple cider vinegar, you're probably eager to start using it. But, before you rush out to grab this miracle product, there are a few things to consider.

Talk with your doctor first. Before you begin using any new health product or start a new health regimen, consult your physician to ensure that there are no risks of that product interfering with current medications, agitating current illnesses, or posing a health risk in any way.

Always dilute it. Because of its high acidity, ACV should never be consumed straight or without dilution to avoid damage to tooth enamel and tissues within the mouth, esophagus, and stomach.

Diabetics, take note! Research suggests that chromium can alter insulin levels. People with diabetes should seek approval from their physician prior to using ACV.

Check bone density. Those who suffer from osteoporosis or already experience low potassium levels should also consult their physicians prior to consuming ACV to ensure that the health benefits of an ACV regimen outweigh any risks.

While most people will never experience any type of harmful side effects by using recommended amounts of ACV, it is important to know the risks

… and recognize that there are still far fewer than many of the seemingly harmless products and medications on the market today.

Chapter 2. Apple Cider Vinegar for Weight Loss

ACV contains enzymes and acids that work to suppress our appetite, leading us to eat less and consume fewer calories. It also has probiotics that helps you burn fat more quickly by speeding up your metabolism. There is also new research showing that ACV can lower blood sugar levels by slowing down the rate at which your body absorbs glucose. That in turn lowers insulin levels which are strongly related to weight loss.

So, if you are thinking about weight loss, then apple cider vinegar provides a natural, home remedy for burning fat, with no bad side effects. In fact, all the side effects of drinking apple cider vinegar for weight loss are good ones - it improves digestion, boosts energy, and strengthens the immune system. Try the following recipes:

SWEET AND SOUR TOFU WITH CACTUS

Ingredients:
- 1Tbs coconut oil
- 1 minced garlic clove
- ½-1tsp ginger, grated
- 1 onion
- 1cup pineapple chunks, canned
- 2Tbs soy sauce,
- Pinch low sodium black pepper
- Thinly sliced cactus leaves
- 3/4 lbs. chunked medium-firm tofu
- 1/4 cup reserved pineapple juice
- 1Tbs of apple cider vinegar
- 1 large thinly sliced carrot

Procedure:
- Remove the eyes and thorns of the cactus leaves.
- Then, heat oil and stir fry the carrots and onions.
- Add in the garlic, the ginger and the cactus leaves and continue to stir fry for 2 minutes.
- Next, add the tofu until it turns golden brown.
- Mix in the rest of the ingredients.
- Cook and wait until they thicken.
- Remove from heat.

- You can get a plate of brown rice and then place one scoop of the mixture on top of the rice.
- Serve and enjoy.

ALMOND FLOUR MUFFINS

Ingredients:
- 1 cup almond flour
- 1 Tbs honey
- ½ tsp apple cider vinegar
- 2 large eggs
- ¼ tsp baking soda
- Muffin pans

Procedure:

- Get a bowl and mix together the baking soda and the almond flour.
- In a separate bowl larger than the first bowl, mix together the eggs and the apple cider vinegar and add the honey as well.
- Then, mix the dry mixture with the wet mixture. Mix them well.
- Next, get a scoop or a spoon and scoop the batter into a muffin pan (each cavity half way). Place the scooped batter onto the baking sheet. Place the pan inside the oven and bake the muffins for 15 minutes at about 350 degrees.
- After 15 minutes, don't remove them from the oven yet but let the muffins cool first.
- Take out the muffins from the oven and serve.

POMEGRANATE VINAIGRETTE

Ingredients:

- 1 large and thinly sliced shallot
- 1 Tbs pomegranate molasses
- 2 Tbs apple cider vinegar
- ½ tsp salt
- ¼ tsp black pepper, freshly ground
- 1/3 cup olive oil

Procedure:

- Mix the pomegranate molasses with the salt, apple cider vinegar, the pepper and the shallot in a bowl.
- Pour in the olive oil and whisk the ingredients together.
- Make sure they are well-mixed until the salt dissolves.
- Serve on top of the salad or serve as a dip.

BRAISED CHICKEN THIGHS WITH APPLE CIDER VINEGAR

- 1Tbs Olive Oil
- Salt and Pepper
- 3 Cloves Minced Garlic
- 1/2 Cup Apple Cider Vinegar
- 1Tbs Butter
- 2 Sliced Carrots
- 1 Sliced Leek
- 1Tbs Flour
- 1-1/2 Cup Chicken Stock
- 4 Chicken Thighs

Procedure:

- First, preheat the oven.
- Then, heat the oil over medium heat in a pot.
- Season the chicken thighs with the salt and the pepper.
- Next, one by one, put them in the pot.
- Cook for about 10 minutes.
- Once cooked, set aside.
- Leave only 1Tbs of oil in the pot and add the garlic, the carrots and the leek.
- Stir occasionally for 5 minutes.
- Add in the flour and wait for a minute.
- Add in the chicken stock.
- Bring to a boil.
- Next, add the chicken thighs into the pot.
- Transfer the pot to the oven and cover it.
- Let it braise for 50 minutes.
- Once braised; transfer to a preheated broiler and broil for a maximum of 6 minutes.
- Remove from the broiler and return the pot to the stove. Cook over medium heat while stirring in the butter. -Serve.

SKINNY ONION RINGS

Ingredients:

- Olive oil spray, extra virgin
- 1/4 cup non-dairy milk
- 1/2 cup brown rice flour
- 1Tbs olive oil, extra-virgin
- 1tsp yeast
- 2 large purple onions
- 2 egg whites
- 1 tsp dill weed
- 1 1/2 cup amaranth, puffed
- 1/4 to1/2 tsp sea salt
- 1/2 tsp curry powder
- 2 Tbs apple cider vinegar

Procedure:

- First, preheat the oven.
- Use the olive oil spray to spray the baking sheet.
- Then, in a bowl, beat the egg whites together with the vinegar, dill weed, the oil, milk and flour. Wait until they are foamy.
- In a separate mixing bowl, mix in the amaranth, the salt and the yeast together. -Next, put the onion rings into the egg white mixture.
- After coating with the egg white mixture, start coating the onion rings again with the dry mixture.
- Spread the coated onion rings onto the baking sheet and bake for 40 minutes. - Serve.

APRICOT SALAD DRESSING

Ingredients:

- ¼ cup olive oil
- 1Tbs apple cider vinegar
- 1 tsp mustard
- 1 tsp lemon juice
- 1 whole fresh apricot, no pits,
- 7 drops of stevia

- ¼ tsp sea salt

Procedure:

- Get a blender place all the ingredients inside it.
- Turn the blender on high setting and blend all the ingredients together until smooth.
- Serve the blended dressing onto your salad or serve as a dip. -Enjoy.

APPLE CIDER VINAIGRETTE

Ingredients:
- 1 cup apple cider vinegar
- 1/2 tsp curry powder
- 1/3 cup half a lemon juice
- 2 tsp seeded mustard
- 1/2 cup fresh and finely chopped chives
- 3/4 cup olive oil, extra-virgin

Procedure:

- Put the apple cider vinegar, the curry powder, the lemon juice, the mustard and the chives into a blender.
- Make sure they are well-blended. Then, add in the olive oil.
- Constantly whisk until well-emulsified. If you wish to add more ingredients, feel free to do so.
- Pour the mixture into a bowl or a dish and serve either with your salad or as a dip.

APPLE CIDER HONEY VINAIGRETTE

Ingredients:

- 1/4 cup apple cider vinegar
- 1 garlic clove
- 1 Tbs dijon mustard
- 2 Tbs fresh lemon juice
- 2 Tbs honey
- 1/3 cup olive oil, extra-virgin
- Salt and pepper to taste

Procedure:

- Stir the mixture well and allow it to marinate for 30-45 minutes before serving.

CUCUMBER SALAD

Ingredients:

- 2 peeled cucumbers
- ½ tsp sea salt
- ½ cup apple cider vinegar

Procedure:

- Slice cucumbers ¼ inch thick.
- Then, place the slices into a bowl. Pour in the apple cider vinegar onto the cucumber slices and sprinkle with salt to season.
- Mix well and serve.

APPLE, WALNUT AND FIG OAT CRISPS

Ingredients:

- 8 peeled, cored and sliced apples
- 1/2 cup brown sugar
- 1 1/2 Tbs apple cider vinegar
- 1 cup flaked rolled oats, small but organic
- 5 Tbs melted butter
- 1/2 cup walnuts, chopped
- 1 cup trimmed and sliced dried figs
- 2 Tbs cornstarch
- 2 Tbs melted butter
- 2 Tbs all-purpose flour
- 1/2 tsp cinnamon, ground
- 4 Tbs crème fraîche

Procedure:

- Mix the apples together with the sugar, vinegar, figs, cornstarch and butter. -Place the mixture in the fridge for an hour. This will make the mixture more flavorful.
- Meanwhile, get a separate bowl and mix in the oats, the butter, the walnuts, the flour and the cinnamon.
- Then, preheat the oven.
- Next, start spreading the apple filling on the bottom. Make sure that the filling is even.
- Pack the filling with oat topping. -Cook this for 45 minutes or wait until the mixture is golden brown.
- Paste a tablespoon of crème fraîche on top and sprinkle with cinnamon. -Serve and enjoy.

CUCUMBER AVOCADO GAZPACHO

Ingredients:

- 1 avocado, small
- 1Tbs minced onion
- 1Tbs lemon juice
- ¼ tsp Celtic sea salt
- 1 cup of water
- 1 peeled and seeded cucumber
- 1Tbs olive oil
- 1Tbs apple cider vinegar
- ¼ tsp chili powder
- Smoked paprika

Procedure:

- Get the blender and mix in the avocado, the onions, the lemon juice the water, the cucumber, the oil and the apple cider vinegar.
- Puree these ingredients on high speed. -Before serving, sprinkle with pepper and salt.

SPICY OVEN FRIES

Ingredients:

- 4 medium potatoes
- 4tsp olive oil, extra virgin
- 2tsp apple-cider vinegar
- 2 1/2Tbs organic ketchup
- 2tsp Worcestershire sauce
- 3/4tsp paprika

Procedure:

- First, preheat the oven.
- Clean the potatoes well and start cutting them into thin strips.
- Then, start combining the ketchup with the sauce, the paprika, the oil and the apple cider vinegar in a large bowl. -Add the potatoes into the ketchup mixture and make sure to coat the potatoes well with the mixture.
- After coating, spread the coated potatoes onto the baking sheet.
- Bake the potatoes for 15 minutes.
- Serve and enjoy.

DATE WALNUT BREAD

Ingredients:

- ½ cup almond flour
- ⅛ tsp sea salt
- 3 large pitted dates
- 1Tbs apple cider vinegar
- 2Tbs coconut flour
- ¼t baking soda
- 3 large eggs
- ½ cup chopped walnuts

Procedure:

- Pulse the two flours together first in a food processor.

- Add in the baking soda and the salt and pulse as well.
- Then, add in the dates and pulse again until coarse.
- Add in the eggs and the apple cider vinegar to pulse as well.
- Pulse the walnuts briefly as well. -Once all these are pulsed, take a loaf pan and transfer this batter. -Put in the oven to bake for 32 minutes maximum.
- Do not remove the pan yet but let the loaf cool inside the oven for at least 2 hours.
- Serve and enjoy.

APPLE CIDER VINEGAR AND HONEY DRINK

INGREDIENTS
- 1 litre water, preferably distilled or filtered
- 2-3 tsp apple cider vinegar, unpasteurized, unfiltered, and organic
- 1 tsp honey
- 1 water bottle

INSTRUCTIONS
- Pour distilled or filtered water into the bottle.
- Shake the bottle of apple cider vinegar well so that the "mother" of vinegar is fully mixed. The mother of vinegar is the most important part of your vinegar since it contains the enzymes and probiotics responsible for the good health reputation of cider vinegar.
- Put 2 to 3 teaspoons of organic ACV in your bottle. Shake the water bottle well so that the vinegar gets all mixed in.
- Now add honey (optional). You can always drink it without. But adding honey improves the taste, especially for those who find the taste of ACV unpleasant. Once you add the honey, shake the bottle well. Your drink is now ready.

WEIGHT LOSS WATER

INGREDIENTS

- 1 tablespoon apple cider vinegar
- 2 cups water
- The juice from ½ of a lemon
- A drop or 2 of raw honey (optional)
- A dash of red pepper (I use Chipotle pepper)
- Ice to taste

INSTRUCTIONS
Mix all ingredients well and enjoy!

IMMUNITY BOOSTER

INGREDIENTS

- 1 teaspoons apple cider vinegar
- 1 cup green tea
- A squeeze of lemon juice
- A drop or 2 of raw honey
- 1 small slice of ginger
- A dash of Ceylon cinnamon

INSTRUCTIONS
- Steep the tea in water for 2-3 minutes.
- Remove tea and stir in the remaining ingredients. *The longer the ginger steeps the stronger it will be.
- Remove ginger slice before drinking.

KICK IT UP SALAD DRESSING

INGREDIENTS
- ½ teaspoon liquid Stevia
- ¼ cup cider vinegar
- ¼ cup extra virgin olive oil
- 1 teaspoon red pepper
- Juice from 1 lemon
- Salt and pepper to taste (you can also use black seeds for the pepper)

INSTRUCTIONS
- Whisk together Stevia, apple cider vinegar, lemon juice and red pepper.
- Slowly pour in olive oil while whisking to emulsify.
- Season with salt and pepper to taste.
- Pour into jar with lid and refrigerate. Makes about ½ cup.

LOSE IT SALAD DRESSING

INGREDIENTS

- ⅓ cup extra virgin olive oil
- 2 tablespoons apple cider vinegar
- 3-4 drops liquid Stevia
- ½ tablespoon Bragg's liquid aminos
- 1 teaspoon finely ground flax seeds
- A dash of salt
- ¼ teaspoon black pepper (you can also use black seeds)
- ¼ teaspoon red pepper
- ½ small clove of garlic, finely grated on a microplane

INSTRUCTIONS

- Whisk together all ingredients until mixed.
- Pour into jar with lid and refrigerate.
- Makes about ⅓ cup.

APPLE CIDER VINEGAR AND GRAPEFRUIT FAT FLUSH

INGREDIENTS

- Apple cider vinegar
- Grape fruit juice
- Oranges
- Honey

DIRECTIONS

In a BPA-free pitcher add the following:
- 1 cup of fresh grapefruit juice
- 1/2 cup of orange juice
- 1 Tbsp Apple cider vinegar
- 1 Tbsp raw honey

You can keep up to 2 days
Drink 2 times a day before a meal.
Make sure all ingredients are organic to get the full health benefits.
Enjoy!

WEIGHT BUSTER

INGREDIENTS

All you need for this simple recipe is a tablespoon of ACV in an 8 ounce glass of water. Drink this before each meal. This is not a miracle drink. It can take up to 4 months before you start seeing real results but hang in there.

Chapter 3. Beauty recipes

TONE YOUR SKIN

If you're one of the many people who spends a pretty penny on top-of-the-line skin toners, you may be relieved to hear that you can instead use apple cider vinegar! When it comes to skin treatments, the same elements that make ACV effective in treating overall health conditions make it an excellent product for treating conditions of the skin as well. The purpose of a skin toner is to remove dead skin cells and oil, refreshing the area of the face and revealing a rejuvenated layer of skin that appears clean, clear, and supple. ACV's vitamins and naturally occurring acids are a safe and effective way to improve the look and feel of skin while also restoring the natural balance of oils and pH of the skin.

TO MAKE A SKIN TONER, COMBINE:

- 1/2 cup warm water
- 1/3 cup ACV
- Few drops of Frankincense essential oil (is a natural skin toner with antibacterial properties)

Soak a cotton ball in the solution and apply directly to the skin of the face and neck. The remaining mixture can be stored in a dark, cool place in an airtight container.

CLEANSE YOUR PORES

Your face is exposed to a number of toxins throughout the day. Airborne elements and tangible dirt and grime adversely affect the appearance and health of your skin. While environmental factors are to blame to an extent, the more common contributor to clogged pores is actually touching your face with your hands—which you likely do dozens of times per day, consciously or subconsciously. When your pores become clogged with unhealthy deposits from your hands, the skin is unable to "breathe" and can develop an oily, greasy, or excessively dry condition.

TO MAKE A PORE CLEANSER, COMBINE IN A BOWL:

- 1/2 cup warm water

- ½ cup ACV
- Few drops of tea tree essential oil (essential for clogged pores and has skin cleaning properties. It will get rid of excess oil that blocks pores)

Use a facecloth to absorb the liquid, ring out the excess, and gently rub the skin with the towel. Repeatedly rinse and reabsorb the ACV mixture, reapplying the mixture to the skin until the skin looks and feels refreshed and clear.

FADE SUNSPOTS

Sunspots appear on the skin in round white patches that may or may not be rough or slightly raised. Long thought to be the result of extensive sun exposure, sunspots are most effectively prevented by reducing the exposure of the skin to the sun's UV rays, wearing clothing to block sunlight from sensitive areas of the skin, and using creams and ointments that prevent sunspots from occurring. While sunlight does aggravate the skin and produce an environment in which sunspots can appear, many medical professionals recommend that sunspot sufferers treat the condition as a fungal infection. For preventive measures, promoting skin cell health and regeneration, and effective antifungal treatments, look no further than apple cider vinegar as an all-encompassing treatment.

The vitamin C present in ACV acts to promote skin health by acting as a powerful antioxidant that can protect skin cells from damage and changes, while also reducing the instance of discoloration on the skin's surface. You can introduce those benefits to your body through this simple drink.

TO MAKE A DRINK, COMBINE:

- 1 cup water or coconut milk
- 1 tablespoon ACV
- 1 teaspoon organic honey

Drink daily. Because of its antifungal properties, ACV has also shown to be effective as a topical treatment for sunspots.

TO MAKE A TOPICAL TREATMENT, COMBINE:

- ¼ cup water
- ¼ cup ACV

Soak a cotton ball or towel in the mixture, and apply directly to the skin for 30 minutes. Repeat this process until the appearance of the sunspots has faded completely.

LESSEN AGE SPOTS

Age spots are brown or tan oval-shaped discolorations on the skin that result from exposure to the sun over long periods of time. These hyperpigmented reactions normally develop in men and women over the age of forty and can become darker and more noticeable as time goes on. While there are chemical treatments and laser treatments designed to whiten these areas and better blend them with surrounding skin tones, many age spot sufferers choose to improve the appearance of their skin through more natural methods such as apple cider vinegar.

With ample amounts of vitamin C and beta carotene that act as powerful antioxidants, apple cider vinegar can assist in the repair of damaged skin cells. In addition to repairing the skin's cells, ACV also acts to regenerate the skin cells and improve the appearance of age spots by renewing the skin's surface.

TO MAKE A TOPICAL AID, COMBINE:

- 1/4 cup ACV
- 1/4 cup water

Apply to the age spots directly on a towelette for 30 minutes three times per day. Many have reported seeing dramatic improvements in the appearance of age spots after a few short weeks of this treatment. In addition, you can also aid the body's reparative systems in regenerating skin cells and fighting free radical damage by consuming a daily ACV drink.

TO MAKE A DRINK, COMBINE:

- 1 cup water
- 1 tablespoon ACV

Drink daily.

MAKE YOUR OWN DEODORANT

Odor on the body can be caused by a number of factors that range from sweat to bacteria, and it is most often strongest in areas of the body that are restricted by clothing or creased, allowing moisture to settle (such as the armpits) where bacteria can thrive. An alarming number of people are unaware that they're placing chemical-laden, store-bought deodorants directly onto a thin layer of skin that covers lymph nodes and veins in the armpit. This highway of blood-transporting veins and nodes absorbs the chemicals and additives in deodorants and antiperspirants and delivers them throughout the body in the blood stream. Because of the possibility of health hazards that can result from the chemicals used in these products, many consumers are opting for natural forms of deodorants that safely and effectively kill the cause of the odor without risking their health.

Apple cider vinegar can be used as an effective deodorant that does not pose health risks and actually boosts the body's overall health.

TO MAKE A HOMEMADE DEODORANT, COMBINE:

- 1 tablespoon water
- 1 tablespoon ACV

Apply the mixture to the armpit or area of odor with a cotton ball and allow to dry. Not only does this application kill odor-causing and infection-breeding bacteria; it is absorbed into the blood stream and helps to assist the body's everyday functioning by ensuring the systems throughout the body receive necessary nutrients.

TO MAKE A PREVENTIVE DRINK, COMBINE:

- 1 cup water
- 1 tablespoon ACV

Drink daily to reap the benefits of health-boosting vitamins, minerals, and antioxidants that prevent odor-causing bacteria from breeding within the body and on the skin's surface.

GET RID OF ACNE

Acne sufferers have long searched for the resolution of blemishes that can appear on the face, neck, chest, back, and arms. Prescription medications and over-the-counter treatments are sometimes expensive, ineffective, or loaded with harsh chemicals and additives. In order to treat the condition safely, naturally, and effectively, acne sufferers can use apple cider vinegar in a number of ways. Apple cider vinegar can be used in four effective treatment options (as a soak, tonic, topical treatment, or facial mask) that are inexpensive, easy to use, and completely risk-free!

TO MAKE A SOAK, COMBINE:

- Tub full of water
- 2–4 cups ACV

Soak for up to 30 minutes.

TO MAKE A TONIC, COMBINE:
- 1 cup water
- 1 tablespoon ACV

Drink daily.

TO MAKE A TOPICAL TREATMENT, COMBINE:
- 1/4 cup ACV
- 1/8 cup water

Apply to skin as needed.

TO MAKE A FACIAL MASK, COMBINE:
1/2 mashed avocado • 1/4 cup ACV
Apply evenly to face, allowing to set for 10 minutes daily.

HAIR TONIC:

2 tablespoons ACV • 1 tablespoon water • 1/2 teaspoon cayenne pepper

Apply directly to the site of thinning hair, rubbing the mixture into the scalp for 5 minutes. Allow it to sit on the scalp for 1 hour before shampooing as usual. You can start to see results within 2–4 weeks. Two chemical compounds in cayenne, capsaicin and quercetin, are the beneficial components that help stimulate hair growth by stimulating hair follicles and improving blood flow of the scalp.

BEAT DANDRUFF

1/2 cup ACV • 1 cup warmed liquid coconut oil

Apply the mixture to the scalp, and allow to sit on the scalp for 30–45 minutes. Rinse before shampooing and conditioning as usual. You can also follow up the ACV and coconut oil treatment with this scalp rinse.

SCALP RINSE:

1/3 cup ACV • 1 cup warm water

Rinse the scalp with the solution after shampooing and conditioning, before towel-drying hair.

MAKE YOUR OWN SHAMPOO

Some shampoos leave you with luscious locks that bounce, shine, and stay frizz-free, while others leave your hair feeling weighed down, dried out, or full of frizz. Trying out different brands can be costly, time-consuming, and damaging to your hair. By using apple cider vinegar as a shampoo alternative, you can naturally cleanse the hair and add beauty and health to your strands. You might even see and feel an improvement in the quality of your hair after just one treatment! ACV is inexpensive, natural, and doesn't contain harsh chemicals and additions (which can actually increase the frequency of bad hair days).

TO MAKE YOUR OWN SHAMPOO:

1/2 cup ACV • 2 tablespoons lemon juice • 1 cup water

Use the mixture in place of your shampoo, massaging it into the scalp and strands, rinsing, and proceeding to condition as you routinely would. You can use this shampoo substitute every wash, or use it alternately with your regular shampoo.

MAKE YOUR OWN CONDITIONER

Nowadays, you can find deep conditioning treatments at home and in the salon, as well as balms and solutions that promise to leave hair silky and hydrated. The variety of conditioning treatments is dizzying. Depending upon whether your hair is oily, dry, curly, or straight, different conditioners designed to treat all hair types may fall flat on delivering their promised results. Surprisingly enough, the same bottle of apple cider vinegar you use for your daily tonics that keep you healthy and energized can also work wonders as a conditioner for hair of all types, shades, and textures. A number of treatment options may be available, but few provide the nutrients contained in ACV, are as inexpensive as ACV, and provide results after the very first treatment like ACV does!

TO MAKE CONDITIONER, COMBINE IN A BOTTLE:

1/2 cup ACV • 1/4 cup liquid coconut oil • 1 cup water

Apply the treatment to your hair, cover hair with a shower cap, and allow the mixture to set for 30 minutes. Then rinse and dry, revealing renewed hair with restored health.

EXFOLIATING APPLESAUCE MASK

INGREDIENTS

- 2 tablespoons organic, preservative free applesauce
- 1 tablespoon ground oats
- 1 teaspoon honey
- 2 teaspoons lemon juice

DIRECTIONS

Combine all ingredients in a bowl and apply to face and neck. Leave on for 10 minutes. As you wash the mask off feel free to gently rub in circular motions. Towel dry and follow with moisturizer.

CLEANSING APPLESAUCE SCALP TREATMENT

INGREDIENTS
- 1/2 cup apple sauce

DIRECTIONS

- Apply organic, preservative free applesauce directly to your scalp and hair. The malic acid will break down any clogged hair follicles and dead skin lingering on the scalp.
- Leave on for 10 minutes and then rinse.

- Conditioner is not necessary as locks will be left shiny and clean.

APPLE CIDER VINEGAR PEEL

INGREDIENTS
- 1 tablespoon organic, raw, unfiltered apple cider vinegar
- 1/2 lemon (optional)

DIRECTIONS
- In a bowl or small cup, pour in the apple cider vinegar and if you are treating pigmentation or sun spots, you can add a squeeze of half a lemon.
- Using a cotton round, dip the cotton in the cup and then gently swab over face in circular motions. Avoid the eye area.
- Tingling sensations are normal, however if you feel burning you can dilute the apple cider vinegar with water.
- Leave the peel on for 5 minutes and then rinse off with warm water

SIMPLE MASK FOR OILY SKIN

INGREDIENTS

- 1 ripe banana
  1 egg white
  1 teaspoon apple cider vinegar or citrus juice

DIRECTIONS

- In a blender, combine the banana, egg white, and vinegar or juice. Blend to form a smooth paste.
- Use a cotton ball to apply the mask to your face, avoiding the eye area. Leave the mask on for 10 to 15 minutes.
- Cleanse thoroughly with warm water, then splash your face with cool water.

LEMON CIDER SCRUB

INGREDIENTS

- 2 Cups Sugar
- 1/4 Cup Coconut Oil
- 1 Tbsp. Lemon Juice
- 1/2 Tbsp. Honey
- 1 Tsp. Apple Cider Vinegar

DIRECTIONS

- Pour sugar into your jar or container, then mix in coconut oil and lemon juice.
- Add honey and apple cider vinegar and mix together for an amazingly fresh body scrub!

ROSE PETAL SCRUB

INGREDIENTS

- 1 cup coconut Oil
- 1/2 cup rose petals
- 1/2 cup raw sugar
- 1/2 cup almond oil

DIRECTIONS

- Pour coconut oil into the jar, then set rose petals on top of the coconut oil and add in sugar.
- Top it off with almond oil, then let the oils soak into the petals. Next, mix it all together and use the scrub on your skin.

FRESH FACE APPLETINI TONER

INGREDIENTS

- 1/2 cup of purified water
- 1/3 cup of apple cider vinegar
- Squeeze of fresh lemon (optional)

DIRECTIONS

- Mix the ingredients in a jar or bottle with a tight-fitting cap.
- After washing your face, shake it up and get your tone on with a cotton ball or piece of soft fabric.
- Follow up with a moisturizer for your skin type. Store the toner in the refrigerator for up to two weeks.

VINEGAR AND HONEY LOTION

INGREDIENTS

- 1 tablespoon honey
- 1/2 teaspoon wheat germ oil or apricot kernel oil Cold-pressed olive oil works too
- 1 teaspoon apple cider vinegar - Cold-pressed and organically grown. We like Bragg's brand—found in health-food stores

DIRECTIONS

- Mix the honey and oil in a bowl until well blended. Then, gradually add apple cider vinegar until you have a pasty consistency.
- Apply the mask and let it stay on your face for 20 minutes. Rinse off with lukewarm water and pat your face

FOOT DEODORIZER

INGREDIENTS

- One cup acv
- Four cups water

DIRECTIONS

- Mix the one-cup apple cider vinegar with four cups water in a basin. Soak feet for 15 minutes, then rinse and dry.
- Apple cider vinegar's antiseptic properties help to deodorize rank odor and disinfect feet. Plus, its anti-fungal attributes prevent and combat fungal conditions like athlete's foot.

Chapter 4. Detoxing

Raw, fermented apple cider vinegar is what you should reach for when you feel the need for a toxin flush. It may be able to improve pH levels and blood sugar levels as well as prevent cancer. In addition, apple cider vinegar may be able to reduce triglyceride levels and protect against Candida infections. Try the following detox recipes:

SUPPER DETOX DRINK

INGREDIENTS
- 1/4 cup apple cider vinegar (raw unfiltered is best-Bragg's brand is great)
- 1/2 teaspoon ground ginger
- 1/2 packet powdered drink mix (I use Designer Whey Tropical Orange Protein 2GO)
- juice of 1-2 lemons
- 1/2 teaspoon stevia (or a few drops liquid stevia)
- 1 quart water

INSTRUCTIONS
- Add all ingredients except water to a cup and whisk to combine completely.
- Mix with water and store in the fridge in a jug or closed bottle.
- When ready to serve, fill a cup halfway with this mixture and dilute with plain water.

GINGER & HONEY SWITCHEL

INGREDIENTS
- 2 inches fresh ginger, grated
- 1/4 cup apple cider vinegar 'from the mother'
- 1 tablespoon honey
- Chilled seltzer
- Fresh mint for garnish

INSTRUCTIONS

Combine grated ginger, apple cider vinegar and honey in a glass. Stir together and chill for 30 minutes. Once chilled, add ice cubes and top with seltzer water - the amount of seltzer you add depends on how diluted you want the drink. Top with fresh mint before serving.

APPLE PIE APPLE CIDER VINEGAR DRINK

Boost your morning with a healthy apple cider vinegar cocktail that tastes like apple pie.

INGREDIENTS
- 2 Tablespoons apple cider vinegar
- 2 Tablespoons no sugar added organic apple juice
- 6 ounces of cold water
- 4 drops of liquid vanilla stevia
- sprinkle of cinnamon
- 1-2 cubes of ice

INSTRUCTIONS
1. Combine all ingredients in a cup and stir or shake to combine. Taste and add more stevia if necessary. Serve chilled or over

MAPLE SYRUP VINEGAR SODA

This simple, vinegared soda is inspired by the drinking vinegars at Pok Pok PDX. Adjust any of the ingredients to suit your preference.

INGREDIENTS
- 1½ tablespoons maple syrup (I prefer Grade B for stronger flavor)
- 1½ tablespoons apple cider vinegar
- ¼ teaspoon vanilla extract
- ¼ teaspoon almond extract
- Approx. 10 ounces cold sparkling water (We use a Sodastream and filtered tap water)
- 3-4 ice cubes

INSTRUCTIONS
1. In a pint glass, mix together the maple syrup, vinegar, and extracts.
2. Fill glass to about 2" beneath the rim with soda water. Stir once gently to combine; being careful not lose too much fizz.
3. Add a few ice cubes to fill remainder of glass. (If you add the ice cubes and then top off with soda water, it may get a bit foamy.)

4. Enjoy!

APPLE CIDER VINEGAR DETOX ELIXIR

INGREDIENTS

- 1 Tbsp raw apple cider vinegar
- 1 Tbsp fresh lemon juice (about 1-2 wedges)
- 1 Tbsp raw honey
- ¼ tsp ginger
- Dash cayenne pepper (seriously just a dash!)

INSTRUCTIONS
1. Mix ingredients in a glass or small jar and add about an ounce of warm water. Drink all at once before eating in the morning.

STRAWBERRY BALSAMIC SHRUB

INGREDIENTS:

- 2 cups strawberries, hulled and quartered
- 1 cup unrefined sugar
- 1 cup apple cider vinegar
- 1 cup balsamic vinegar

DIRECTIONS:

- In a medium bowl with a lid, sprinkle the sugar over the already hulled and quartered strawberries.
- Put the lid on the bowl and set aside in the refrigerator for 2 days.
- When removing strawberry and sugar mixture from the refrigerator you will notice that a syrup has formed and the strawberries have turned to mush. This is perfect!
- Using a strainer, strain the syrup away from the strawberries into another bowl.
- Press on the strawberries using a spatula to remove all excess syrup. Remove leftover sugar with a spoon and scoop into the bowl with the remaining syrup. You don't want to waste that sugar!
- Discard the mushy strawberries once all of the retained syrup is removed from them.
- Add both the apple cider vinegar and the balsamic vinegar to the bowl and stir. Using a small funnel, pour the syrup and sugar into

a glass bottle with a cap. Set in the refrigerator for another 2-3 days or until all of the sugar is fully dissolved.

STRAWBERRY SHRUB SYRUP RECIPE

INGREDIENTS

- 1 cup fresh strawberries, hulled and quartered
- 1 cup white sugar
- 1 cup cider vinegar

DIRECTIONS

- In a glass bowl, mix together strawberries and sugar.
- Cover and refrigerate for 1-3 days.
- Strain out strawberry pieces from the syrup using a fine mesh sieve.
- Mix cider vinegar and strawberry syrup and pour into a mason jar. Store shrub syrup in the refrigerator.

STRAWBERRY SHRUB COOLERS

Mix 1/4 cup shrub syrup with 1/2 cup seltzer water and pour into an ice filled glass. Enjoy!

APPLE SHRUB RECIPE

INGREDIENTS

- 1 1/4 cups grated SweeTango or Honeycrisp apples
- 3/4 cup organic cane sugar
- 1 cup raw apple cider vinegar

DIRECTIONS

- Add apples, sugar, and apple cider vinegar to a glass mason jar. Attach jar cover tightly and shake liberally.
- Refrigerate and let sit for 3-4 days.
- Remove from refrigerator and strain juice into a large bowl, then squeeze remaining juice out of apples using a colander.
- Pour juice into a glass container and keep refrigerated.
- Will stay good for up to 6 months if stored properly in refrigerator.

PEACH SHRUB

INGREDIENTS
- 1 cup peeled and chopped peaches (I used an assortment of yellow and white)
- 1 cup organic sugar
- ½ cup apple cider vinegar
- ½ cup white wine vinegar

INSTRUCTIONS
- Combine the peeled and chopped peaches with the sugar, cover, and let macerate for 24-36 hours, stirring periodically. (I let them sit in the fridge, but you can start with 1-2 hours out on the counter to accelerate the process.)
- Add the vinegars, stir, mash the fruit a bit, cover, and let sit at room temperature for a few hours to be sure the remaining sugar dissolves, stirring periodically.
- Once the sugar is dissolved, mash the fruit some more, re-cover and place in the refrigerator for about a week, stirring twice a day.
- Strain out the peach pieces over a clean jar, pushing down on them to release as much juice as possible. Discard the solids (or use as you see fit--they're basically pickled at this point).
- Cover tightly and mark the date, so you don't forget. The shrub should be able to be stored in the refrigerator safely for several months.

GORGEOUS VERY BERRY SMOOTHIE RECIPE

INGREDIENTS

- 1 16oz bag of frozen mixed berries (strawberries, blackberries, blueberries, and raspberries)
- 1 banana
- 2 cups almond milk (might need more, depending upon consistency desired)
- 2 scoops vanilla protein powder (I use Spirutein)
- 2 tbsp apple cider vinegar
- a dash or two of fresh ground Himalayan sea salt

INSTRUCTIONS

- Combine all ingredients into a blender; mix well.
- Add more almond milk as needed to reach desired consistency (some like it thicker than others)

DIY EUCALYPTUS AND VANILLA BATH SALTS

INGREDIENTS:

- 1 cup Epsom salt
- 1/2 cup baking soda
- 3 drops eucalyptus essential oil
- 8 drops vanilla in jojoba oil
- Green food coloring (optional)

DIRECTIONS:

- Add the Epsom salt, baking soda and essential oils to a large sealable plastic bag.
- If you are using food coloring to give the bath salts a hue, add one drop to the ingredients in the plastic bag.
- Seal the bag closed and use your hands to massage the contents so the food coloring mixes in with the ingredients.
- Transfer from the plastic bag to a glass container with a lid.
- Use one spoonful per bath.

GINGER DETOX BODY SCRUB

INGREDIENTS

- 1 tablespoon fresh ginger
- ½ cup of Epsom salt
- 1 tablespoon lemon juice

INSTRUCTIONS

- Combine roughly chopped ginger and ½ cup Epsom salt in a food processor. Pulse a few times until the ginger is ground and combined.
- Remove to a small bowl and add lemon juice.
- Put down a towel and apply scrub before your detox bath

BACK PAIN BATH SALTS

INGREDIENTS

- 2 cups Epsom salts
- 1 cup bi-carb soda
- 10 drops peppermint essential oil
- 5 drops eucalyptus essential oil
- 5 drops rosemary essential oil
- 5 drops lavender essential oil
- 5 drops cinnamon essential oil
- 2 tbsp dried lavender flowers
- 1 tbsp fresh rosemary sprigs

INSTRUCTIONS

- Mix together Epsom salts and bi-carb soda in a large bowl. Add essential oils and stir well to distribute evenly through salts. Gently stir through dried lavender flowers and rosemary sprigs.
- Transfer salts into glass jar/s. Use 1 cup of bath salts per bath and soak for at least 15 minutes.

DIY CALMING & DETOXING BATH SALTS

INGREDIENTS

- 1 1/2 cups dead sea salts
- 1/2 cup cup epsom salt
- 1/2 cup real salt
- 1/8 cup bentonite clay
- 7 drops lavender essential oil
- 7 drops frankincense essential oil

INSTRUCTIONS

- In a glass mixing bowl, combine all ingredients and mix with a non-metal spoon {metal can destroy the healing properties of the clay}.

- Store in an air-tight glass jar.

BATH INSTRUCTIONS

- Add 1 cup of bath salts mixture to a hot bath. Don't add bubbles or soap to the water.
- Relax and soak for 15-20 minutes so your body can sweat, detox and absorb all of the nutrients.
- When you're ready to get out of the tub, rinse off with water {not soap} if you chose.

LEMON ROSEMARY BATH SALTS

INGREDIENTS:

- 2 cups epsom salt
- 1/2 cup baking soda
- 2-3 tbsp fresh rosemary; finely chopped
- 6-8 drops lemon essential oil
- 2-3 tbsp lemon zest (optional)

DIRECTIONS

- In a bowl combine epsom salt and baking soda. Add in half of the essential oil drops, mix, then add in the remaining drops.
- Mix in the chopped rosemary and lemon zest if you decide to use it until fully combined.
- Store in an airtight container.

LAVENDER DETOX BATH RECIPE:

INGREDIENTS:

- 1 cup Epsom Salt
- 1 cup Baking Soda
- 10 drops of Lavender Essential oils

DIRECTIONS:

1. Pour contents into hot bath water and soak for 20 minutes. Try to cover your entire body up to your neck.
2. Once you get out of bath, avoid eating anything for 20 minutes and

drink plenty of cold water.

LAVENDER EUCALYPTUS BATH SOAK

INGREDIENTS
- 2 cups Epsom Salts
- 1/2 cup dry lavender
- 5-6 drops pure lavender essential oil
- 10 drops pure eucalyptus essential oil

INSTRUCTIONS
- Combine all ingredients in a small bowl, fill bathtub with very warm water, add the combined ingredients, and soak for about 20 to 30 minutes.
- Word of caution: before getting up take a couple deep breaths to allow oxygen back to the brain, and get up slowly. Epson Salts can make you feel a little lightheaded if not used to regular soaks.

ALMOND MILK BATH RECIPE

INGREDIENTS
- 1 cup epsom salts
- 1/2 cup baking soda
- 1/2 cup Silk Almondmilk
- 2 tablespoons coconut oil
- 10-15 drops of essential oil

INSTRUCTIONS
- Mix ingredients together then add to a warm bath as the water is running.
Enjoy your bath for at least 20 minutes.

BAKING SODA DETOX BATH

INGREDIENTS
- 1 Cup of Epsom salt
- 2 Cup of **Baking soda**

INSTRUCTIONS

- Combine 1-part Epsom salt to a 2-part baking soda – mixture creates this basic detox bath for one 30 minute soak. For a *first detox bath*, measure 1 cup of Epsom salt and 2 cups of baking soda.
- Add mixture while drawing hot bath water, filling the tub 2/3 of the way full.
- Soak for at least one half hour.

SEA SALT DETOX BATH

Ingredients

- 1/3 Cup **Epsom salts**
- 1/3 Cup Sea salt
- 1/3 Cup **Baking soda**
- 2 1/2 tsp **Ground ginger**
- 1 Cup **Apple cider vinegar**

Instructions

- Combine all of the dry ingredients in a bowl.
- Draw a bath with hot water, as hot as you handle. As the water is filling the tub, add all of the dry ingredients and the vinegar. The flowing water will help mix it, but make sure to mix it up well. (If your water turns yellow or orange, that's just the ginger and the vinegar).
- Soak for about 40 minutes and relax.

Chapter 5. Breakfast, lunch, dinner, salads and salad dressings

APPLE CIDER VINEGAR BREAKFAST BREW

INGREDIENTS

- 1/4 cup water
- 1/4 cup unfiltered apple cider vinegar
- 1 tablespoon honey
- 1 teaspoon cayenne pepper
- 1 wedge lemon

DIRECTIONS

- Bring water to a boil.
- Combine hot water and apple cider vinegar in a small glass or mug.
- Add honey and cayenne pepper. Stir well. Top off with a squeeze of lemon.
- Take a deep breath of the mixture, and start drinking.

SPRING BREAKFAST SALAD

INGREDIENTS
- 2 tbsp pancetta, cooked and crumbled
- 8 asparagus spears, blanched
- Large handful baby spinach
- Large handful arugula
- 4 cremini or baby bella mushrooms, sliced very thinly
- 2 tbsp very thinly sliced red onion
- 2 tbsp shaved parmesan
- 1/4 cup savory granola
- 2 eggs, poached or fried over-easy

DRESSING:

- 1 tsp maple syrup
- 1 1/2 tsp olive oil
- 1 1/2 tsp apple cider vinegar
- Pinch salt and freshly cracked black pepper

INSTRUCTIONS

- Cook pancetta in a small skillet. Drain and set aside.
- Wash a cut asparagus into 2-inch pieces. Boil 2 cups of water in a saucepan. Add asparagus spears and boil for 1 minute until bright green. Remove asparagus with a slotted spoon and immediately place into a bowl of ice water to stop cooking process. Drain.
- Whisk dressing ingredients in a small bowl.
- In a large bowl, combine spinach, arugula, mushrooms, onions, and asparagus. Add dressing and toss it all together. Divide between two plates or bowls. Top each with granola, pancetta, and parmesan.
- Use same pot of boiling water to poach eggs: Add a splash of vinegar to gently boiling water. Using slotted spoon, stir water rapidly in a circle to create a swirling motion with water. Gently crack eggs, one at a time into boiling swirling water. Cover and let cook for about 1 minute for a runny yolk or 2-3 minutes for a more solid yolk. Remove eggs from water with slotted spoon.
- Place a poached egg on top of each salad and serve immediately

APPLE CIDER COFFEE CAKE

INGREDIENTS
- 1 cup almond meal (almond flour)
- 1/4 cup coconut flour
- 1/3 cup applesauce (regular or unsweetened)
- 1 oz dried apple (chopped)
- 50 grams Vanilla protein powder (about 2 scoops)
- 2 tbsp Raw Apple Cider Vinegar
- 1/4 tsp sea salt
- 1/2 tbsp nutmeg, ginger, and clove combined (or just one if you don't have both)
- 1/2 tsp cream of tartar
- 1/2 tsp baking powder
- 2 eggs
- 1 tsp liquid stevia (optional)
- To make it sweeter add 2-3 tbsp honey (optional)

- butter or coconut butter
- Note: You don't have to use protein powder. But it does give it bulk. Sub any other flour there (about 1/4 cup). If you like it more dry, then take out the applesauce.

INSTRUCTIONS

- Mix your flour and dry ingredients first. Set aside. Whisk your egg and then fold in the Grain free flours. Add the applesauce and dried apple and mix again. Pour into a greased bread pan (i used 9×9) or brownie pan.
- Bake at 350F for 15-16 minutes or so. Remove from oven and pour a little melted butter or coconut butter on top, then let it cool.
- This bread is lightly sour and sweet. If you want it to be sweeter, add in more stevia. It's great with yogurt or cream cheese!

APPLE, WHITE CHEDDAR, AND SPINACH SALAD WITH HONEY-APPLE CIDER VINAIGRETTE

INGREDIENTS:

Salad
- about 6 cups fresh spinach
- 1 large apple, cored and sliced very thin (try Envy, Gala, Fuji, or similar)
- 1 cup grated aged white cheddar
- 1/2 cup dried orange-flavored cranberries (I use Trader Joe's; plain dried cranberries may be substituted)
- 1/2 cup Fisher Natural Sliced Almonds
- Honey-Apple Cider Vinaigrette
- 1/4 cup olive oil
- 1/4 cup honey
- 1/4 cup apple cider vinegar
- 2 teaspoons mustard (I like either dijon or honey mustard)
- 3/4 teaspoon salt, or to taste
- 3/4 teaspoon black pepper, or to taste

DIRECTIONS:

- **Salad** - To a large bowl or platter, add all ingredients in the order listed; set aside.
- **Honey-Apple Cider Vinaigrette** - In a small glass jar or container with a lid, add all ingredients, put the lid on and shake vigorously

until combined; taste vinaigrette and tweak as necessary to taste. Drizzle over salad, toss to combine, and serve immediately. If you don't use all the vinaigrette, extra will keep airtight in the fridge for up to 1 week.

PAN COOKED CHICKEN & APPLE

INGREDIENTS
- 2 boneless chicken breasts
- 1 splash EVOO oil
- 1 onion, chopped
- 3 clove garlic, minced
- 2 apples, cored and sliced
- ¼ cup apple cider vinegar
- 2 Tbsp honey mustard
- 1 handful fresh sage leaves

INSTRUCTIONS
- Start with some oil in a pan, heat on medium-hot then add the chicken breast. Cook chicken breast for 5 minutes on each side, browning then nicely but not cooking them all the way through.
- Remove the chicken from the pan to a plate, lower heat to medium and sauté half of a chopped onion and 3-4 minced garlic cloves for a few minutes then add 2 peeled, cored and sliced apples, 1/4 cup of cider vinegar, 1 tvsp of honey mustard, and a couple tbsps of fresh sage.
- After about five minutes add chicken back into the pan with everything else. Cover with a lid tightly. Let it simmer at low-medium for 10-15 minutes or until chicken is fully cooked.

CREAMY TUNA PASTA SALAD WITH GREEK YOGURT

INGREDIENTS
- 1/2 of 13 oz package of whole wheat rotini (or pasta of your choice)
- 2 cans light tuna, drained and flaked
- 3 hard boiled eggs, chopped
- 3 celery stalks, chopped (include celery leaves for more flavor)
- 1/2 cup plain 0% Greek Yogurt
- 1 tablespoon light mayo (optional, can use more Greek yogurt instead)
- 1 tablespoon mustard

- 1 1/2 teaspoon lemon pepper seasoning (I use a no salt added seasoning, check yours and adjust your additional salt)
- 1/8 teaspoon onion powder
- couple of splashes of apple cider vinegar (I measured a cap full)
- salt and pepper to taste

DIRECTIONS

- Prepare your pasta according to directions. When cooked through, drain and set aside to cool.
- To a large bowl add tuna, hard boiled eggs and celery.
- Prepare your "dressing" by combining Greek yogurt, mayo, mustard, lemon pepper, onion powder, apple cider vinegar, salt and pepper.
- Add your cooled pasta to large bowl along with your dressing. Gently stir to combine. Taste for salt and pepper and adjust.

SLOW-COOKER PULLED PORK SANDWICHES

INGREDIENTS

- 3 Tbsp light brown sugar
- 2 tsp hot paprika
- 1 tsp mustard powder
- ½ tsp ground cumin
- Kosher salt and freshly ground pepper
- 1 (3- to 4-lb) boneless pork shoulder, trimmed of excess fat
- 2 tsp vegetable oil
- ½ cup apple cider vinegar, plus more to taste
- 3 Tbsp tomato paste
- 6 potato buns

Barbecue sauce and prepared coleslaw, for serving

DIRECTIONS

- Combine 1 tablespoon brown sugar, the paprika, mustard powder, cumin, 2 teaspoons salt and 1/2 teaspoon pepper in a small bowl. Rub the spice mixture all over the pork.
- Heat the vegetable oil in a large skillet; add the pork and cook, turning, until browned on all sides, 5 minutes. Remove the pork and transfer to a plate; whisk 3/4 cup water into the drippings in the skillet. Transfer the liquid to a 5-to-6-quart slow cooker.
- Add the vinegar, tomato paste, the remaining 2 tablespoons brown sugar and 2 cups water to the slow cooker and whisk to combine.

Add the pork, cover and cook on low, 8 hours.
- Remove the pork and transfer to a cutting board. Strain the liquid into a saucepan, bring to a boil and cook until reduced by half, about 10 minutes. Season with salt. Roughly chop the pork and mix in a bowl with 1 cup of the reduced cooking liquid, and salt and vinegar to taste. Serve on buns with barbecue sauce and coleslaw.

HOMEMADE SLOPPY JOES

INGREDIENTS
- 1¼ to 1½ lbs ground beef
- half of a small onion, finely chopped
- half of a small green pepper, finely chopped
- ¼ teaspoon garlic powder
- 1 cup ketchup
- 2 tablespoons brown sugar
- 2 teaspoons yellow mustard
- 1 tablespoon apple cider vinegar
- 1 tablespoon soy sauce

INSTRUCTIONS
- Brown onions and green peppers with ground beef over medium heat until meat is cooked through and vegetables are soft. Drain meat and return to pan.
- Add garlic powder, ketchup, brown sugar, mustard, vinegar, and soy sauce. Mix well and simmer for 5 to 10 minutes.
- Serve on soft hamburger buns.

SALT AND VINEGAR SQUASH CHIPS

INGREDIENTS
- 1 yellow squash or zucchini (2 cups)
- 2 teaspoons olive oil
- 2 tablespoons Bragg's apple cider vinegar
- salt

INSTRUCTIONS
- Slice squash on mandoline at 1/8 setting (or, if you want thicker chips, a higher setting).

- Mix olive oil, vinegar, and salt. Put squash in and mix around to coat.
- Put squash slices on Teflon sheets on dehydrator trays.
- Dehydrate at 110º for 12 hours or until crispy.

APPLE CIDER VINEGAR AND SAGE CHICKEN

Yields: 4 serving

INGREDIENTS

- 4 chicken breasts, bone in and skin on
- 2 cups organic chicken stock
- 1 ¼ cups organic apple cider vinegar
- 3 onions, thinly sliced
- 4 tablespoons extra virgin olive oil
- 3 tablespoons sage, chopped
- 3 tablespoons honey
- 4 garlic cloves, chopped
- Juice of ½ a lemon
- Salt and pepper to taste

DIRECTIONS:

- Preheat a Dutch oven over a medium-high heat.
- Add two tablespoons of olive oil to the pan.
- Season chicken with salt and pepper, then add them to the hot oil, skin side down.
- Brown the chicken for about 5 minutes per side, then remove them from the pan and set them aside for later.
- Add another 2 tablespoons of olive oil to the pan, then add the onion slices, sage, honey, and the garlic.
- Season the onions with salt and pepper and cook over a medium-low heat, stirring frequently for about 20 minutes or until the onions are really brown and starting to caramelize.
- Add the apple cider vinegar to deglaze the pan, taking care to scrape up all the brown bits on the bottom of the pan with a wooden spoon.

- Now add the chicken stock and heat the mixture until it starts to bubble.
- Once at a rolling simmer, return the chicken to the pot with the liquid and onions.
- Place a lid on the pot, turn the heat to medium and simmer for about 20 minutes, turning the chicken over in the sauce about halfway through the cooking time.
- When the 20 minutes is up, remove the lid and check to make sure the chicken is cooked through by cutting a small slit in the thickest part of the breast with a paring knife to have a look inside. If it is cooked through the juices will run clear and the meat will be white not pink.
- Remove the chicken to a plate, squeeze over the lemon juice, and cover with foil to keep warm.
- Turn the heat of the sauce up to high and simmer until the sauce thickens up slightly, about 4–5 minutes.
- Serve the chicken drizzled with the sauce and your favorite side dish of vegetables or a healthy salad.
- Dig in!

APPLE CIDER VINEGAR PORK CHOPS

Yields: 6 servings

INGREDIENTS:
- 6 pork chops
- 2 cups unsweetened apple juice
- ¼ cup organic apple cider vinegar
- ¼ cup finely chopped onion
- 1 tablespoon olive oil
- 1 tablespoon butter
- 1 tablespoon Dijon mustard
- 1 tablespoon minced sage
- ¼ teaspoon red pepper flakes
- 4 garlic cloves, minced
- Salt and pepper to taste

DIRECTIONS:

- Heat the oil and butter in a large non-stick pan over a medium heat and brown the pork chops on both sides. Transfer the pork chops to a plate.
- Now add the onion and garlic to the pan and cook until they start to brown.
- Now pour in the apple juice and apple cider vinegar and scrape up all the browned bits with a wooden spoon.
- Add the mustard, stir, and bring to a boil.
- Once boiling, reduce the heat and cook until the sauce thickens, about 5 minutes.
- Stir in the rosemary and red pepper flakes, then return the chops to the pan and heat them through.
- Season with salt and pepper and then serve with your favorite side dish.
- Enjoy!

BATTERED CAULIFLOWER WITH TANGY TOMATO DIPPING SAUCE

Yields: 2 servings

INGREDIENTS:

For the Batter:
- ¾ cup rice flour
- ¾ cup sparkling water
- ½ cup corn starch (or substitute tapioca)
- ¼ teaspoon baking soda
- Pinch of salt

For the Sauce:
- 2 cups mixed peppers, chopped (red, green, yellow, and orange)
- 1 red onion, chopped
- ¼ cup cashews, roughly chopped
- ¼ cup tomato paste, no added sugar
- 4 tablespoons coconut aminos
- 4 tablespoons organic or homemade vegetable stock
- 2 tablespoons organic apple cider vinegar
- 1 tablespoon fresh ginger, grated
- 1 tablespoon garlic, minced

- 2 teaspoons Stevia
- 1 teaspoon sesame oil
- 1 teaspoon red pepper flakes

OTHER INGREDIENTS:
- 2 pounds cauliflower, cut into small florets
- ¾ cup rice flour

DIRECTIONS:

- Preheat the oven to 400°F.
- First prepare your batter: mix all the batter ingredients together until they are smooth. Place in the fridge to chill.
- Boil your cauliflower florets in some lightly salted water for about 5 minutes or until they are just beginning to soften. Drain and then pour cold water over them to stop the cooking process. Set them aside to cool.
- Place the rice flour into a resealable bag and add the cooled cauliflower pieces. Gently shake the bag to coat the cauliflower in the rice flour.
- Dip each floret into the chilled batter, then place the cauliflower onto a parchment lined baking tray and bake for 10 minutes, then turn them over and bake for another 10 minutes. The cauliflower is cooked when it has a crunchy golden crust.
- Remove the cauliflower to a plate to cool down and make the sauce.
- Heat up the sesame oil in a large non-stick pan and add the peppers, onion, ginger, and garlic. Cook until the onions and peppers are soft, then add the rest of the ingredients and stir together well.
- Bring the sauce to a boil, stirring constantly, then remove from the heat and add the cauliflower.
- Totally YUM!

BRAISED CHICKEN THIGHS

Yields: 2 servings

INGREDIENTS:
- 6 chicken thighs, bone in, skin on

- 2 cups organic or homemade chicken stock
- ½ cup organic apple cider vinegar
- ¼ cup celery, chopped
- 2 carrots, peeled and sliced
- 1 leek, sliced
- 1 onion, chopped
- 4 garlic cloves, minced
- 1 tablespoon butter
- 1 tablespoon olive oil
- 1 tablespoon plain flour
- Salt and pepper to taste

DIRECTIONS:

- Heat the olive oil up in a Dutch oven, then place the chicken pieces in skin side down and cook until the skin is golden-brown and crispy.
- Remove the chicken from the pot and drain off most of the oil, leaving about 1 tablespoon, then add the onions, carrots, celery, garlic, and leek and cook until they begin to soften, stirring often.
- Stir in the flour and cook for a further 2 minutes, then deglaze the pan with the apple cider vinegar. Take care to scrape up all the bits of browned chicken off the bottom of the pan, then pour in the stock and bring it all to a boil.
- Once boiling, add the chicken back to the pot, skin side up.
- Cover the Dutch oven and place it into a 350°F oven for 1 hour.
- When the cooking time is up, place the chicken pieces onto a baking tray and pop them under the broiler so that the skin can crisp up again.
- While the chicken cooks, place the pot onto the stove and allow the sauce to reduce and thicken over a medium heat, then stir in the butter.
- Serve the chicken slathered in delicious sauce with your choice of sides.
- Enjoy!

BRAISED PORK CASSEROLE

Yields: 4 servings

INGREDIENTS:

- 2 ½ pounds pork shoulder, trimmed of excess fat and cut into cubes
- 2 onions, chopped
- 2 cups unsweetened apple juice
- ¾ cup organic apple cider vinegar
- 2 tablespoons olive oil
- 2 tablespoons fresh sage, chopped
- 1 tablespoon butter
- 2 bay leaves
- 2 garlic cloves, minced
- Salt and pepper to taste

DIRECTIONS:

- Place an oven-proof casserole dish over a high heat on the stove.
- Add half the butter and half the oil and brown the pork in batches, placing them onto a plate when they are done.
- Add the rest of the butter and the oil and brown the onions and garlic.
- Pour the apple juice and apple cider vinegar into the pan to deglaze, carefully scraping all the browned bits off the bottom of the pan with a wooden spoon.
- Place the pork back into the pan along with the rest of the ingredients and bring it to a simmer.
- Once simmering, place the whole dish into an oven preheated to 325°F and cook uncovered for 1 hour or until the meat is tender and the cooking liquid has reduced.
- Serve hot with some rice.
- Delicious!

COUSCOUS SALAD

INGREDIENTS
- 2 cups water
- 2 cups couscous
- 1 pound butternut squash, cut into strips
- 1 red pepper, seeds removed and cut into quarters
- 2 onions, peeled and quartered
- ¼ cup fresh parsley, chopped
- 3 tablespoons organic apple cider vinegar
- 6 tablespoons olive oil
- 3 tablespoons sesame seeds
- 1 tablespoon soy sauce
- 1 teaspoon garlic salt, or to taste
- Salt and freshly ground black pepper to taste

DIRECTIONS
- Toss the squash, red pepper, and onions with 3 tablespoons of olive oil and the garlic salt and roast in the oven at 350°F for 30 minutes or until they are tender and browning.
- Remove from the oven and set aside. When the veggies are cool enough to handle, you can chop the red pepper and onion up into bite sized pieces.
- While the veggies roast, make the couscous. In a medium saucepan, bring the water to a boil, then stir in the couscous
- Cover, remove from the heat, and let stand for about 5 minutes or until all the water has been absorbed.
- Combine the apple cider vinegar, salt, pepper, and soy sauce in a small bowl and set aside.
- Sauté the sesame seeds in the remaining olive oil over a low heat for a minute or two until they just start to brown.
- Remove from the heat. Add the vinegar and soy sauce mixture and stir together well.
- Fluff the couscous lightly with a fork and break up any clumps.
- Combine the couscous, roasted vegetables, and chopped parsley, then toss everything to mix.
- Pour over the sesame seed, vinegar, and soy sauce mixture and toss again.
- If you like, you can add a little more salt to taste and garnish with more chopped parsley.
- Serve warm or chilled.

- Out of this world!

GERMAN POTATO SALAD

INGREDIENTS
- 4 pounds potatoes (about 8 cups sliced)
- 3 cups onion, chopped
- ¾ cup organic apple cider vinegar
- ¾ cup hot water
- ¼ cup organic bacon, cooked and diced
- 2 tablespoons raw organic honey or maple syrup
- 2 tablespoons chives, chopped
- Sea salt and pepper to taste

DIRECTIONS
- Boil the potatoes until tender.
- Peel and slice them while warm.
- Add the onions, honey, or maple syrup, bacon, salt, and pepper and toss gently.
- Mix the apple cider vinegar mixed with the hot water, then pour the mixture over the potatoes, bacon, and onions.
- Toss together lightly so as not to break up the potatoes too much.
- Sprinkle with the chopped chives for garnish.
- This salad can be served warm or cold—either way it is delicious!

KALE AND AVOCADO SALAD

INGREDIENTS:
- 1 bunch organic kale, stems removed
- 1 avocado, cut into bite-sized cubes
- 8 ounces organic cherry tomatoes, halved
- ¼ cup red onion, sliced
- ¼ cup sunflower seeds
- 1 tablespoon raw honey
- 1 tablespoon olive oil
- ¼ cup organic apple cider vinegar
- Pinch of sea salt

- Juice of ½ a lemon

DIRECTIONS:

- Tear the kale into bite-sized pieces and place them into a large salad bowl.
- Prepare the vinaigrette by blending the honey, olive oil, vinegar, salt, and lemon juice in a blender until well combined.
- Pour the vinaigrette over the kale and massage well until the kale has softened.
- Top with the avocado cubes, red onion, cherry tomatoes, and sunflower seeds.
- Serve immediately and enjoy!

MIXED MARINATED BEANS

Yields: 10 servings

INGREDIENTS

- 1 pound frozen green beans, cooked and drained
- 1 pound canned kidney beans, drained
- 1 pound canned wax beans, drained
- 1 onion, thinly sliced
- 1 green bell pepper, chopped
- 1 cup cherry tomatoes, sliced
- ¾ cup organic apple cider vinegar
- ¼ cup raw organic honey (optional)
- ½ cup olive oil
- 1 teaspoon garlic, minced
- ½ teaspoon salt
- ½ teaspoon freshly ground black pepper

DIRECTIONS

- Combine the drained beans in a large bowl with the sliced onion, sliced cherry tomatoes, and bell peppers.
- Mix the vinegar, honey, olive oil, garlic, salt, and black pepper in a jar, put the lid on and shake well.
- Pour the mixture over the beans and toss well to combine.
- Cover the bowl and marinate overnight in the refrigerator.

- Serve when needed with your favorite meat dish.
- YUM!

HOMEMADE SALAD DRESSING

INGREDIENTS:
- ½ cup olive oil
- ⅓ cup organic apple cider vinegar
- ¼ teaspoon salt
- 1 teaspoon raw organic honey or maple syrup (optional)
- 1 garlic clove, crushed
- ½ teaspoon dry mustard
- ½ teaspoon paprika
- ¼ teaspoon black pepper

DIRECTIONS:

- Combine all the ingredients in a jar, shake, and serve. *Do not refrigerate.*

MAYONNAISE

Yields: 4 servings

INGREDIENTS:
- 1 cup olive oil
- 1 cup macadamia oil
- 5 egg yolks, at room temperature
- 1 tablespoon organic apple cider vinegar
- 1 tablespoon Dijon mustard
- Salt and pepper to taste

DIRECTIONS:

- Add everything to the blender except for the oils and blend until well incorporated.
- Now very slowly, a drop at a time, add the olive oil, while the blender runs continuously.

- Keep adding the olive oil slowly until it starts to emulsify, then add the macadamia oil and keep blending until it is all incorporated.
- Store in the fridge for 1 week.

Chapter 6. Natural Cures Healing the Body of Disorders

IMPROVING IMMUNITY

Ingredients:

- 1 teaspoon of apple cider vinegar
- 1 cup of green tea
- A few drops of pure lemon juice
- 2 to 3 drops of raw honey
- 1 small slice of raw ginger
- A pinch of cinnamon

Directions:

Allow this to steep in hot water for 2 to 3 minutes before drinking. Don't forget to remove the ginger before drinking.

GETTING RID OF GALLSTONES

If you are having a gallstone attack, you need to mix 1 tbs of apple cider vinegar in a cup of apple juice. To get rid of gallstones, drink no more than 2 tsp of ACV in a glass of water 3 times a day before each meal.

ACID REFLUX:

The majority of people in our society suffer from acid reflux. You will need to mix 2 tsp of ACV in a glass of water before meals.

DANDRUFF AND HAIR LOSS:

Apply an equal amount of apple cider vinegar and water to a spray bottle. Spray your hair and scalp before shampooing and conditioning.

ACUTE SINUS INFECTION:

Mix 8 ounces of warm water to 2 tablespoons of apple cider vinegar, as well as a few drops of honey. Also, add 1/8 of a cup of apple cider vinegar in a vaporizer.

HIGH BLOOD PRESSURE:

You will need 2 tablespoons of ACV in a glass of water daily. Do this for 30 days!

HICK UP CURE:

You will need:

1/4 tsp shot of ACV straight.

Keep in mind that in the long run this can burn the esophagus but for a short term miracle cure try it. You'll be thankful you did.

FOR CHEST CONGESTION:

Cut open a paper bag and make it into a sheet the size of your chest. Soak this sheet in ACV. Sprinkle one side with black pepper. Apply it across your chest for about a half hour.

COLD AND FLU

A body that's alkaline is more effective at fighting off viruses, flu's and colds. Add 2 teaspoons of apple cider vinegar to warm water or hot tea. Do this just before a cold starts to set in. If you are already very sick, keep drinking ACV, it will still help your body fight off any infection or germs. It will improve your overall health and give you energy as well.

NATURAL TEETH WHITENER

One of my apple cider vinegar uses is as a natural teeth whitener. Take your finger and rub apple cider vinegar on your teeth for 1 minute. Then rinse mouth out with water. The pH of apple cider vinegar can remove stains from your teeth which helps naturally whiten.

CAN KILL CANDIDA (YEAST) AND BOOST PROBIOTICS

Millions of people around the world struggle with candida and yeast. The side effects can be bad breath, lack of energy, UTI's and digestive issues. ACV contains probiotics and a type of acid that promotes the growth of probiotics which help kill off candida. Remove sugar from your diet and consume 1 tbsp of apple cider vinegar 3x daily as part of a candida cleanse.

REGULATES YOUR BODIES PH

Apple cider vinegar contains acetic acid which is acidic in nature but has a more alkaline effect on the rest of your body. Balancing your bodies pH can reduce your risk of chronic illnesses like cancer and can dramatically increase your energy.

AN ALL-NATURAL HOUSEHOLD CLEANER

The anti-bacterial properties and the balanced pH of apple cider vinegar make it a perfect household cleaning product. Fill a spray bottle with 50% water and 50% ACV then spray windows and counters for cleaning.

BALANCES BLOOD SUGAR AND IMPROVES DIABETES

Medical research has proven that the acetic acid found in apple cider vinegar can balance blood sugar and improve diabetes. Put apple cider vinegar on salads or consume 1 tablespoon in water before meals.

HEAL POISON IVY

The minerals in apple cider vinegar like potassium can help reduce swelling and inflammation, improving poison ivy. Also, ACV can help detox the poison out of your skin helping poison ivy heal more quickly.

REPEL FLEAS ON YOUR PETS

Mix a 50/50 solution of apple cider vinegar together and soak your pet in a tub. Do this 1x a day for several weeks to rid your pet of a flea infestation.

FIGHT SEASONAL ALLERGIES

Another amazing treatment of ACV is for allergies. ACV helps break up mucous in your body and support lymphatic drainage. It also supports the immune system and can clear your sinuses. Put 2 tablespoons in a large glass of water and drink 3x daily for allergies.

KILL FUNGUS ON TOES AND SKIN

The anti-bacterial and anti-fungal compounds in apple cider vinegar make it a great natural cure for skin and toenail fungus. Simply rub on the area of fungus 2x daily. Also, using a mixture of coconut oil and oil of oregano is great for killing fungus.

EASE VARICOSE VEINS

Apple cider vinegar is excellent for varicose veins because it improves circulation in the vein walls and is anti-inflammatory so reduces bulging veins. Combine apple cider vinegar with witch hazel and rub on veins in circular motion and you should see improvements in two weeks.

ACV CURES WARTS

Put apple cider vinegar topically on wart and then cover in band aide or bandage. Leave on overnight and remove in the morning. You may see results in one week or it could take longer. Thousands have sworn that apple cider vinegar cured warts and other skin issues

ACV CAN BE USED AS A NATURAL AFTERSHAVE.

Fill a bottle with equal parts apple cider vinegar and water, and shake before applying to the face.

CONCLUSION

Apple cider vinegar truly is a magical elixir. There can be no downside to including it in your daily diet. So welcome health, beauty, and vitality into your life with as little as a tablespoon of this amazing liquid a day. There is no part of your body that is excluded from enjoying the miraculous benefits of apple cider vinegar, literally from top to toe, inside and outside; your body can enjoy something positive when you use it regularly.

So don't waste another minute—welcome apple cider vinegar into your life today! You won't regret it!

More Health Books:

Salad Dressing Recipes: The World's Best Organic Gluten Free Salad Dressing Cookbook Recipes
By Alicia Hern

https://www.amazon.com/Salad-Dressing-Recipes-Organic-Cookbook-ebook/dp/B01LW7LIXZ/ref=sr_1_1?ie=UTF8&qid=1483916293&sr=8-1&keywords=salad+dressing+recipes+alicia+hern

Donut Cookbook: 20 Organic Gluten Free Donut Recipes
By Dina Sheppard

https://www.amazon.com/Donut-Cookbook-Organic-Gluten-Recipes/dp/1530745047/ref=sr_1_18?ie=UTF8&qid=1483915658&sr=8-18&keywords=donut+cookbook

Fruit Salad Recipes: 20 Organic Gluten Free Fruit Salad Cookbook Recipes
By Rebecca Lei

https://www.amazon.com/Fruit-Salad-Recipes-Organic-Cookbook/dp/1537602543/ref=sr_1_41?ie=UTF8&qid=1483915888&sr=8-41&keywords=fruit+salad+recipes

Gluten Free Cupcakes: My Sweet Little Gluten Free Cupcake Cookbook

By Lindsey Moore

https://www.amazon.com/Gluten-Free-Cupcakes-Cupcake-Cookbook/dp/1536809152/ref=sr_1_5?ie=UTF8&qid=1483916011&sr=8-5&keywords=gluten+free+cupcakes

Natural DIY Makeup and Cosmetics Books

DIY Makeup And Homemade Beauty Products

By Julia Broderick

https://www.amazon.com/DIY-Makeup-Homemade-Beauty-Products/dp/1523264160/ref=sr_1_1?ie=UTF8&qid=1483827055&sr=8-1&keywords=diy+makeup

Homemade Beauty Products

By Elina Grace

https://www.amazon.com/Homemade-Beauty-Products-Formulating-Chemical/dp/1532942273/ref=sr_1_9?ie=UTF8&qid=1483827055&sr=8-9&keywords=diy+makeup

DIY Makeup: The Beginner's Guide To Formulating Natural Cosmetics

By Sandra Lei

https://www.amazon.com/DIY-Makeup-Beginners-Formulating-

Cosmetics/dp/1523390557/ref=sr_1_10?
ie=UTF8&qid=1483827055&sr=8-10&keywords=diy+makeup

DIY Makeup: Making Natural Cosmetics And Creating Homemade Beauty Products For The Modern Woman

By Melina Houston

https://www.amazon.com/DIY-Makeup-Cosmetics-Creating-Formulating/dp/1535485450/ref=sr_1_14?
ie=UTF8&qid=1483827055&sr=8-14&keywords=diy+makeup

Homemade Beauty Products: Making Natural Cosmetics And DIY Makeup

By Serena Phan

https://www.amazon.com/Homemade-Beauty-Products-Natural-Cosmetics/dp/1523322993/ref=sr_1_23?
ie=UTF8&qid=1483827114&sr=8-23&keywords=diy+makeup

DIY Makeup: The Art Of Making Natural Cosmetics

By Rose De Lena

https://www.amazon.com/DIY-Makeup-Making-Natural-Cosmetics-ebook/dp/B01D0PJN0O/ref=sr_1_24?
ie=UTF8&qid=1483827141&sr=8-24&keywords=diy+makeup

DIY Makeup: The Goddess Guide To Creating All Natural Homemade Beauty Products

By Isabella Dalia

https://www.amazon.com/DIY-Makeup-Creating-Formulating-Cosmetics-ebook/dp/B01D6NA9CQ/ref=sr_1_33?ie=UTF8&qid=1483827167&sr=8-33&keywords=diy+makeup

Homemade Lip Balm: Fun And Unique DIY Lipstick And Lip Balm Recipes

By Mandy Phan

https://www.amazon.com/Homemade-Lip-Balm-Lipstick-Recipes/dp/1535545984/ref=sr_1_38?ie=UTF8&qid=1483827189&sr=8-38&keywords=diy+makeup

Homemade Makeup: Formulating Natural Cosmetics

By Audrey Silva

https://www.amazon.com/Homemade-Makeup-Formulating-Natural-Cosmetics-ebook/dp/B01APYF884/ref=sr_1_4?ie=UTF8&qid=1483827232&sr=8-4&keywords=homemade+makeup

Printed in Great Britain
by Amazon